How to Eat to Modify Your Drinking

Change Your Relationship with Alcohol by Healing Your Gut, Healing Your Mind, and Improving Your Nutrition

Michael M. Gagne

Contents

Introduction

An individual's eating habits not only have a substantial impact on their overall health, but they also have the potential to affect how they interact with alcohol. A multidimensional approach that includes nutrition, psychology, and physiology is required to gain an understanding of how different dietary choices can be used to influence drinking habits. Through an examination of the relationship between the intake of food and alcohol, this book will provide insights into the process of making educated decisions to support a healthier lifestyle.

The Connection Between Consuming Alcohol and Dieting:

It is vital to recognize the physiological and psychological connections between drinking habits and food to have a complete understanding of how food influences drinking habits. Diets that are high in nutrients can improve mental health and mood, which may in turn reduce the desire to experiment with alcohol as a kind of self-medication. Poor nutrition and diets that are not balanced can, on the other hand, be a contributor to tension and anxiety, which in turn increases the possibility of turning to alcohol as a means of relieving stress and anxiety.

Macronutrients in a Balanced State: How your body reacts to alcohol might be affected by the nature of the foods you consume. The management of macronutrients, which include carbs, lipids, and proteins, might be of critical importance. Protein-rich diets help balance blood sugar levels, minimizing the probability of cravings and impulsive drinking. Healthy fats, such as those found in avocados and almonds, contribute to satiety, limiting excessive alcohol consumption. Complex carbs give a sustained flow of energy, increasing general well-being and maybe minimizing the dependency on alcohol for a rapid energy boost.

Hydration and alcohol consumption: Proper hydration is crucial to a healthy lifestyle and can also affect drinking habits. Drinking water consistently helps maintain good bodily processes and can act as an alternative to alcoholic beverages in social circumstances. Moreover, staying hydrated helps minimize the intensity of hangovers, deterring excessive alcohol intake the night before.

Mindful Eating and Drinking: Mindful eating entails paying attention to the flavors, textures, and sensations of each bite, and building a better relationship with food. Applying this notion to drinking can raise awareness of alcohol usage. Enjoying alcoholic beverages consciously, and appreciating each sip, may lead to a more modest intake. Combining mindful eating and drinking can offer a holistic approach to general well-being.

Nutrients That Support Mental Health: Certain nutrients play a key role in maintaining mental health, and adding them to your diet may positively influence your drinking behavior. Omega-3 fatty acids, present in fish and flaxseeds, have been associated with enhanced mood and reduced impulsivity, potentially moderating the desire to overindulge in alcohol. Additionally, meals high in vitamins B and D contribute to general mental well-being, building a foundation for better decisions.

Alcohol and Blood Sugar Levels: Understanding the impact of alcohol on blood sugar levels is crucial for making informed dietary decisions. Consuming alcohol can lead to variations in blood sugar, thus triggering cravings for sweet foods. Opting for balanced meals that help control blood sugar can attenuate these desires and lessen the chance of excessive alcohol consumption.

Foods That Support Liver Health:

The liver plays a vital role in digesting alcohol, making its health crucial in controlling drinking behaviors. Incorporating foods that support liver function, such as cruciferous vegetables, berries, and green tea, can help with general well-being and potentially lessen the risk of alcohol-related liver disorders.

Social Influences and Dietary Choices:

Social circumstances often involve the intake of alcohol, making it vital to balance peer pressure and societal standards. Making conscientious nutritional choices in social contexts might influence not only your relationship with food but also your

alcohol consumption. Opting for non-alcoholic alternatives or setting personal limitations can help maintain a balanced approach to socializing without relying on alcohol as a social lubricant.
Seeking professional guidance:
While dietary improvements might positively affect drinking behaviors, it's vital to recognize when professional aid is needed. Individuals battling with alcohol dependence or having difficulty reducing their consumption should seek help from healthcare professionals or addiction specialists. A holistic strategy combining nutrition, therapy, and medical assistance may be important for long-term success.

PART 1

Evaluating The Need For Change In Your Relationship With Alcohol

The relationship people have with alcohol in today's culture is a complicated and multidimensional part of who they are. Some use it as a way to celebrate, relax after a hard day, or act as social glue. For others, though, this relationship may develop into something more troublesome, with a range of negative social, emotional, and physical effects. Fostering a healthier lifestyle requires being aware of the warning signs and determining whether changes in one's alcoholic relationship are necessary.

Comprehending the connection: Since alcohol is frequently embedded in social and cultural contexts, it is initially safe to consume in moderation. But when the distinction between excess and moderation gets hazy, it can be a sign of a developing problem. Think about analyzing your drinking habits, comprehending the causes of your alcohol intake, and determining whether it has changed from a choice to a compulsion.

Physical and psychological effects: Drinking too much alcohol can have negative effects on one's physical and emotional health. It's critical to pay attention to any changes in your health, like exhaustion, weight swings, and disturbed sleep patterns. Assess your mental state as well; chronic mood swings, increased irritation, or a growing reliance on alcohol as a stress reliever could be signs of trouble in a relationship.

Social Structure:

An individual's social interactions can be greatly impacted by their relationship with alcohol. Consider whether drinking has taken center stage in your social life and affected your relationships with friends and family. It may be time to reevaluate the role alcohol plays in your life if drinking becomes a

bigger part of social events or if people start to worry about your conduct.

Effect on Accountabilities:

A dysfunctional alcoholic relationship's interference with day-to-day tasks is one of its main indicators. Consider whether your drinking has caused you to overlook your personal, professional, or family responsibilities. When drinking starts to interfere with your capacity to perform your duties, it's time to consider how your lifestyle and the substance are balanced.

Identifying a Pattern:

Behavior patterns frequently reveal information about the character of a person's relationship with alcohol. Cravings that cause you to lose focus or the inability to regularly follow self-imposed boundaries could be indicators of an unhealthy pattern. It is essential to identify and deal with these tendencies to start a constructive shift.

Evaluating Reliance:

Alcoholism can take many different forms, from urges that are physical to an emotional dependence on the drink. Determine whether cutting back or giving up feels onerous or unachievable. If you experience anxiety or distress when you consider giving up alcohol, this could be a sign of a dependency that needs to be addressed.

Looking for assistance:

Changing your alcoholic relationship frequently requires outside assistance. Reaching out to others can offer helpful viewpoints and support, whether via friends, family, or professional advice. A support system, therapy, or counseling can help you work through the difficulties of changing your relationship with alcohol.

Examining other options:

Consider change as a chance to investigate healthier options rather than as a sign of deprivation. Develop new interests, take part in fulfilling activities, and surround yourself with people who share your desire for positive change. The path to a more harmonious and healthy relationship with alcohol is restoring happiness and contentment in life. Assessing if your alcoholic relationship needs to change is a complex and unique process. It requires self-reflection, pattern recognition, and a readiness to ask for help. Although implementing a change could be difficult, there are incalculable advantages for your social, mental, and physical health. Through proactive measures and cultivating an attentive mindset, you can start a transforming path toward a better relationship with alcohol.

1. To **Drink or Not To Drink**

A Personal Reflection on the Choice of Alcohol Consumption. In a society where social events typically concentrate around the clinking of glasses and the shared enjoyment of alcoholic beverages, the decision of whether to join in drinking is a very personal one. The choice to use alcohol is impacted by several factors, including cultural conventions, individual values, health considerations, and personal experiences. As one navigates through life, the dilemma of whether to drink or not becomes a constant topic, stimulating contemplation and self-exploration. Alcohol has been a fundamental component of human history, ingrained in cultural customs and rituals across civilizations. From the ancient libations presented to deities to the toasts hoisted in contemporary celebrations, the significance of alcohol is apparent. However, as society's opinions toward alcohol evolve, so does the individual's consideration of its significance in their own life. One's upbringing typically impacts their outlook on drinking. Some individuals grow up in circumstances where alcohol is regarded with reverence and moderation, developing a healthy relationship with its intake. Others may have observed the adverse impacts of heavy drinking within their family, leading to a more cautious approach. Childhood experiences, whether happy or unpleasant, leave an everlasting impression on one's attitude toward alcohol and contribute to the ongoing internal conversation about whether to embrace or avoid it. Cultural influences play a key role in establishing attitudes about alcohol intake. In some communities, drinking is a fundamental aspect of socializing and bonding. Festivals, weddings, and other joyful occasions are typically accompanied by the clink of glasses and the shared enjoyment of alcoholic beverages. For people engaged in such societies, the decision to abstain may be viewed with curiosity or even opposition. Conversely, in societies that promote temperance, choosing not to drink may be more socially acceptable, if not expected. The media also plays a vital role in affecting opinions about alcohol. Advertisements and portrayals of drinking in film and television typically romanticize the experience, portraying it as an integral component of a luxurious existence. These images can establish unreasonable expectations and contribute to the urge to indulge in social drinking. On the other hand, the media also sheds light on the darker side of alcohol usage, exposing its potential for abuse and related health hazards. Balancing these competing messages becomes a difficulty for anyone attempting to make educated decisions about their relationship with alcohol. Personal values and beliefs significantly complicate the decision-making process. For some, the choice to refrain from alcohol accords with sincerely held ideals, whether anchored in religious views, personal health concerns, or a commitment to maintaining clarity of mind. Others may consider alcohol a form of relaxation and social lubrication, leading them to adopt it into their lives in moderation. The interplay between individual ideals and society's expectations forms a complicated tapestry that determines one's position on alcohol intake. Health factors add another element of complication to the decision-making process. The potential health advantages and hazards connected with alcohol intake have been the subject of substantial research and controversy. While moderate alcohol intake has been linked to certain cardiovascular advantages, excessive drinking has major health hazards, including liver disease, addiction, and greater vulnerability to accidents. Individuals must weigh these considerations against their personal health situation and make informed decisions that accord with their well-being. Personal experiences with alcohol, whether favorable or unpleasant, have a key role in shaping one's relationship with it. Positive encounters may build a sense of camaraderie and satisfaction, promoting the belief that alcohol may be a joyful and sociable lubricant. Conversely, unpleasant experiences, such as witnessing the ill effects of drunkenness or experiencing personal harm, may serve as warning tales, motivating a more careful approach or even complete abstinence.

Potential risks associated with alcohol consumption?

The National Institute on Alcohol Abuse and Alcoholism states that excessive alcohol use can have detrimental effects on one's health. The following are some dangers connected to using alcohol in excess:

Brain: Alcohol can alter how the brain functions and appears by interfering with its communication networks. These disturbances can alter behavior and mood, as well as impair cognition and coordination.

Heart: Drinking excessively over an extended period or all at once can harm the heart, leading to issues such as cardiomyopathy: heart muscle elongation and drooping rhythm abnormalities in the heartbeat; a stroke of high blood pressure.

Liver: Excessive alcohol use damages the liver and can cause several issues and inflammations in the liver, such as fatty liver or steatosis. Alcohol fibrosis and cirrhosis causes hepatitis.

Pancreas: Drinking alcohol makes the pancreas create harmful chemicals that might eventually develop pancreatitis, a hazardous inflammation that can cause the organ to enlarge, hurt, and perhaps spread while also impairing the organ's capacity to produce hormones and enzymes necessary for healthy digestion.

Cancer: The National Cancer Institute states that there is substantial scientific evidence linking alcohol consumption to

several cancer forms. There are now
unmistakable trends linking alcohol use
to higher risks of some cancer types:
head and neck cancer, including oral
cavity, pharynx, and larynx malignancies.
stomach cancer, especially stomach
squamous cell carcinoma. Carcinoma of
the liver. Carcinoma of the breast. Colon
cancer.
It's crucial to know the possible
advantages and hazards of alcohol
consumption and to drink in moderation.
It's wise to seek advice from a healthcare
provider if you're not sure whether to
drink or not.

1. The Dr. and the Wine Bottle

Once upon a time, in the lovely hamlet of
Vinopolis, there lived a great physician
named Dr. Evelyn Merlot. In addition to
her medical knowledge, Dr. Merlot was

highly regarded for her profound taste in excellent wines. Vinopolis, a city renowned for its wineries and vineyards, offered the ideal setting for Dr. Merlot to pursue his two interests, enology and therapy.

Shelves crammed with medical papers gave way to an unexpected assortment of wine bottles in Dr. Merlot's office. Every bottle contained a narrative, a remembrance of a patient whose life she had impacted, or shared a happy moment upon a successful diagnosis. The strange relationship between the doctor and her wine collection was a topic of frequent whispers in the town.

A strange patient showed up at Dr. Merlot's office one day. The patient was a gloomy, shadowy figure whose symptoms confused even the seasoned physician. Dr. Merlot was determined to solve the mystery, so he thoroughly examined the patient and reviewed their medical history. But advancement remained elusive.

Dr. Merlot was drawn to her collection of wine bottles during a reflective time. She looked at the labels; each one described a different grape kind, aging method, and flavor character. It was at this contemplative moment that she understood the bond between her patients and the wines she loved.

This realization gave Dr. Merlot the idea to combine her passion for wine with medicine. She started looking into wine's possible medical advantages, not as a treatment but rather as an adjunct to a whole-health strategy. Dr. Merlot found that moderation and mindfulness were important while studying the historical practices around the medical use of wine. In her clinic, she began holding special sessions where patients were asked to tell their stories over thoughtfully chosen wines. The environment turned friendly and supportive, fostering a place where healing transcended the material world. Some colleagues expressed skepticism towards Dr. Merlot's nontraditional approach, but her patients reported significant improvements in their overall health.

The patient in the shadows changed with the seasons. With the help of Dr. Merlot's creative techniques, the enigmatic person started to reveal herself gradually but steadily. The therapeutic power of the shared stories and the carefully designed wine experiences proved profound. The illness, which had hitherto been a mystery, began to come to light.

In addition to being a very accomplished doctor, Dr. Merlot gained recognition as a pioneer in integrative medicine. She wrote papers, gave talks, and even worked with wineries to investigate the possibilities of medicinal combinations. Vinopolis developed as a gathering place for those looking for unusual but successful wellness strategies.

The pivotal moment occurred when Dr. Merlot accepted an invitation to speak at the town's annual wine festival. She described her voyage of discovery while standing on stage amid the vines and bottles, which represent her passions. Despite their initial skepticism, the audience paid close attention as she discussed the significant link between responsible wine use and healing.

Beyond Vinopolis, Dr. Merlot's method became well-known in the years that followed. Her creative techniques made their way into mainstream treatment, and medical organizations welcomed the incorporation of holistic practices. After making a full recovery, the once-mysterious patient started advocating for the healing potential of fusing mindfulness with medicine.

The story of Dr. Merlot and the wine bottle came to represent the endless opportunities that arise when curiosity, enthusiasm, and open-mindedness come together. Vinopolis, which was eternally altered by the physician's spirit of innovation, lived on as a shining example of cutting-edge medical care and a love of better things in life.

2. The Trilogy of Drinking Patterns

Drinking habits weave a complicated tale in the delicate tapestry of human behavior, reflecting not just personal preferences but also cultural conventions, psychological dynamics, and societal influences. Three separate phases comprise the trio of drinking habits, which are beginning, moderation, and escalation. Each step develops a distinct story, highlighting the varied ways in which individuals connect with alcohol.

Starting Point:

The initiation phase, which is defined by the discovery of alcohol, is covered in the first chapter of the trilogy. It frequently starts while people are navigating their newfound freedoms and social expectations during the adolescent-to-adult transition. Many people start drinking because of peer pressure, curiosity, and the need to fit in. Experimentation, when people test the limits of alcohol use and determine their tolerance levels, is what defines initiation.

Social and cultural factors are crucial in determining drinking habits throughout this stage. Alcohol is frequently used at social events, holidays, and milestones in life, normalizing its presence in a variety of contexts. A person's connection with alcohol is built during the initiation phase when habits are established that may last a lifetime.

Moderation in action:

The moderation phase assumes a significant role as the story moves further. Drinking at this stage is done in moderation and under control. People going through this stage frequently have a positive relationship with alcohol, allowing it to be a part of their lives without taking over. To consume alcohol in moderation, one must be aware of both its possible drawbacks and advantages. During the moderation phase, social and cultural influences continue to impact drinking habits. Acceptable alcohol consumption amounts are set by social norms, and responsible drinking is frequently recommended. But the border between moderation and excess can be thin, and people may find themselves living on the brink when their circumstances and outside influences change.

Increase in severity:

The trilogy's last act takes place during the escalation phase when drinking habits become increasingly dangerous. A rise in alcohol consumption frequency and volume is indicative of an escalation. What was once a way to unwind or a social glue can become a coping strategy or a means of escaping the difficulties of life.

Drinking habits might worsen as a result of psychological variables like stress, trauma, or mental health conditions. Genetics might also be involved since certain people are more likely than others to form unhealthy interactions with alcohol. Several negative outcomes, such as deteriorated relationships, physical health problems, and decreased functioning in several spheres of life, can result from escalation.

The three drinking habits together provide a complex picture of how people behave when they consume alcohol. Every person has a different path through these phases, which go from the initiation phase, which is characterized by curiosity and social exploration, to the moderation phase, which is characterized by balance and control, and the escalation phase, which is when patterns grow more complicated and perhaps harmful. Gaining knowledge of these drinking habits can help us better understand the larger societal forces that influence how we see alcohol. It makes people think about how society's expectations, cultural norms, and individual experiences affect the decisions people make about drinking alcohol. We may better comprehend the nuances of the human experience with alcohol by dissecting the three drinking patterns. This opens the door to more intelligent treatments, support networks, and dialogues.

PART 2

A Practical Method For Maintaining Sobriety

For those in recovery from addiction, maintaining sober is a difficult but transformative path. An approachable strategy for attaining and maintaining sobriety is examined in this note. It includes a holistic strategy that attends to mental, emotional, and physical health. Through the integration of multiple treatments, individuals can establish a strong basis for long-term recovery.

Understanding Triggers: A key component of the sobriety path is the ability to identify and comprehend triggers. Acknowledging circumstances, feelings, or persons that could trigger a relapse enables people to create coping strategies. This entails introspection and therapy to identify the root causes of addiction.

Creating a Support System: It's critical to have a strong support system in place. Having a supportive network of friends, family, or support groups around oneself helps one stay accountable and encourage one another. Having regular conversations with these people can help them emotionally when things are hard.

Attending Therapy: Getting professional therapy, such as group and individual counseling, is essential to sustaining recovery. Therapeutic methods support people in addressing co-occurring mental health conditions, learning coping mechanisms, and investigating the underlying reasons for addiction.

Taking Up a Healthy Lifestyle: Mental and physical health are related. Overall well-being is improved by leading a healthy lifestyle that incorporates frequent exercise, a well-balanced diet, and enough sleep. Particularly exercise has been shown to release endorphins, which have been shown to improve mood and lessen cravings.

The integration of mindfulness and meditation techniques can assist in stress management and the development of self-awareness. By encouraging people to live in the present, these techniques lessen the chance that they will give in to temptations or triggers.

Setting Achievable Short- and Long-Term Goals: Having realistic goals gives you direction and a sense of purpose. These objectives ought to be quantifiable, reasonable, and flexible enough to change as conditions do. No matter how tiny the milestone, celebrating it encourages healthy behavior.

Creating Hobbies and Interests: Distracting attention and energy from desires can be achieved by partaking in rewarding and pleasurable activities. Interests and hobbies provide people with a sense of fulfillment and success, which enhances their general sense of well-being.

Self-Education: Information is a valuable aid in the healing process. Acquiring knowledge about addiction, its consequences, and different approaches to treatment enables people to make wise choices. Understanding the significance of continuous self-improvement is facilitated by education as well.

Sustaining Routine and Structure: Creating a daily schedule and preserving order give stability. Regular timetables foster a sober environment by lowering uncertainty and anxiety. In order to end the cycle of addiction, consistency is essential.

Celebrating Progress: A good outlook is fostered by recognizing and appreciating one's own accomplishments. Acknowledging progress strengthens the resolve to live a sober lifestyle, whether it's reaching a personal goal, finishing a recovery milestone, or staying sober for a set amount of time.

Remaining sober is a complex process that calls for commitment and a thorough strategy. People can build a strong basis for long-lasting recovery by integrating self-awareness, support networks, treatment, a healthy lifestyle, mindfulness exercises, goal-setting, hobbies, education, and structure. This useful technique is a framework that may be tailored to specific needs and situations rather than a one-size-fits-all answer. With the correct resources and attitude, people can successfully navigate the route of sobriety and achieve a satisfying, drug-free existence.

3. Alcohol and Nutrition: A Changing Relationship

For many years, the connection between alcohol intake and nutrition has been a subject of discussion. New findings and viewpoints have helped to clarify the intricate interactions between the two. The complex interactions between alcohol and nutrition are examined in this note, along with how cultural changes, scientific discoveries, and societal views have influenced our perception of them.

Historical Background:

Alcohol has always played a significant role in many different civilizations and societies. Alcohol has been used in a variety of contexts, from prehistoric ceremonies to contemporary social events. However, past perspectives on nutrition frequently concentrated on the calorie content of alcohol rather than its nutritional value. Alcoholic drinks were historically viewed as an energy source with minimal regard for their nutritional content.

Shifting Viewpoints:
There has been a change in perception of alcohol's nutritional effects in recent years. Research has challenged preconceived notions by highlighting both positive and negative elements. While some cardiovascular advantages have been linked to moderate alcohol consumption, excessive drinking can have negative effects on general health. Assessing the nutritional effects of alcohol requires an understanding of the thin line that separates moderation from excess.

Macronutrients and Caloric Content:
Drinking alcohol increases the amount of calories consumed each day by a large amount. But these calories frequently

don't contain important nutrients, which raises questions about "empty calories." Moreover, alcohol's metabolism differs from that of other macronutrients, which can have an impact on the body's energy balance and even lead to weight gain. Alcohol's effects on the absorption and use of nutrients are a complicated topic that needs more research.

Minerals and vitamins:
Drinking alcohol can affect how well the body absorbs and uses vitamins and minerals. Long-term alcohol consumption can cause shortages of important nutrients like zinc, folic acid, and vitamin B12. These inadequacies may have far-reaching effects, impairing several body processes and accelerating the emergence of health problems.

Liver Purpose:
The liver is essential for the metabolism of alcohol and the digestion of nutrients. Overindulgence in alcohol can damage

the liver and make it more difficult for it to properly process nutrients. This may lead to dietary deficits and jeopardize general health. Evaluating the wider nutritional impact of alcohol requires an understanding of the complex link between alcohol and liver function.

Social and Cultural Factors:

Alcohol consumption and diet are highly influenced by social and cultural factors. Diverse drinking habits, societal expectations, and cultural customs influence people's views toward alcohol use. Furthermore, the social context of drinking frequently entails dietary decisions that go along with it, which further affects the nutritional impact overall.

Implications for Public Health:

There are significant ramifications for public health from the evolving link between alcohol and nutrition. Promoting informed decision-making requires educating the public about the possible drawbacks and advantages of alcohol use. Initiatives in the field of public health should not only focus on the nutritional side of alcohol consumption but also its wider effects on general health.

Drinking alcohol can harm your health in several ways. The National Institute on Alcohol Abuse and Alcoholism states that excessive alcohol use can result in the following health issues:

Brain: Alcohol can alter how the brain functions and appears by interfering with its communication networks. These disturbances can alter behavior and mood, as well as impair cognition and coordination.

Heart: Drinking excessively over an extended period or all at once can harm the heart, leading to issues such as hypertension, arrhythmias (an irregular heartbeat), cardiomyopathy (the stretching and sagging of the heart muscle), and stroke.

Liver: Heavy drinking takes a toll on the liver and can lead to a range of disorders and liver inflammations, including steatosis, fatty liver, alcoholic hepatitis, fibrosis, and cirrhosis.

Pancreas: Drinking alcohol makes the pancreas create harmful chemicals that might eventually develop pancreatitis, a hazardous inflammation that can cause the organ to enlarge, hurt, and perhaps spread while also impairing the organ's capacity to produce hormones and enzymes necessary for healthy digestion.

Cancer: Drinking alcohol is known to cause cancer in humans and can lead to several different types of cancer. Drinking alcohol has been linked to higher chances of head and neck cancer, esophageal cancer, liver cancer, breast cancer, and colorectal cancer, among other cancers.

It's crucial to remember that alcohol has more detrimental impacts on health than just those listed above. The World Health Organization has also established a connection between alcohol use and serious noncommunicable diseases such as liver cirrhosis, some types of cancer, and cardiovascular diseases, as well as mental and behavioral disorders like alcoholism.

Three types of liver disease can be caused by excessive alcohol consumption: alcoholic hepatitis, which is an **inflammation of the liver;** fatty liver, which is an excessive accumulation of fat in the liver, and alcohol-related cirrhosis, which is the replacement of normal liver tissue with scar tissue. The first stage of alcohol-related liver disease, fatty liver, affects almost all heavy drinkers. Although they may have an enlarged liver or experience mild discomfort in the upper right side of the abdomen, most people with fatty livers may not exhibit any symptoms.

Drinking alcohol can harm your health in several ways. The National Institute on Alcohol Abuse and Alcoholism states that excessive alcohol use can result in the **following health issues:**

Brain: Alcohol can alter how the brain functions and appears by interfering with its communication networks. These disturbances can alter behavior and mood, as well as impair cognition and coordination.

The brain's neurotransmitters, which are chemical messengers that send information throughout the body and are largely responsible for regulating behavior, emotion, and physical activity, are affected by alcohol consumption. Drinking causes the neurotransmitter

GABA to slow down, which causes drunk people to move slowly, speak slurredly, and react slowly. Alcohol also accelerates the release of glutamate, a neurotransmitter that controls dopamine in the brain's reward region. Pleasure and well-being are produced by this.

4. Hormones and Blood Sugar Regulation

Controlling blood sugar levels is essential for preserving general well-being and health. The complex interaction between hormones and other physiological processes is essential for maintaining strict control over blood glucose levels. This paper examines the major hormones that control blood sugar, their roles, and the complex feedback loops that support glucose homeostasis.

Insulin

The pancreatic beta cells that produce insulin are the main hormones involved in controlling blood sugar levels. Insulin is released when blood glucose levels rise, such as following a meal, to help cells absorb glucose. To be stored in the muscles and liver, this hormone encourages the conversion of glucose into glycogen. Insulin also prevents the liver's process of gluconeogenesis, which produces glucose from non-carbohydrate sources.

Glucagon:

In contrast to insulin, the pancreatic alpha cells create glucagon. Glucagon is released when blood glucose levels fall, which can happen during physical exercise or in between meals. This hormone causes the liver to release glucose into the bloodstream by converting stored glycogen into glucose. In addition, glucagon stimulates the production of gluconeogenesis, which raises blood sugar and meets the body's energy needs.

Cortisol:

The adrenal glands generate cortisol, sometimes known as the stress hormone. Although its main function is in reaction to stress, cortisol also plays a part in blood sugar control. It encourages the production of gluconeogenesis, which guarantees a continuous supply of glucose during times of high stress or extended fasting. On the other hand, persistently high cortisol levels may cause insulin resistance and contribute to long-term blood sugar abnormalities.

Both norepinephrine and epinephrine The hormones known as "fight-or-flight" are norepinephrine and adrenaline, which are produced by the adrenal glands. These hormones are released during stressful situations or emergencies, setting off a series of reactions that make sure the body is ready for rapid action.

One of its effects is to boost blood sugar levels by accelerating glycogen breakdown in the liver and promoting gluc *we*ose release into the bloodstream.

hormones of the thyroid:

Thyroxine (T4) and triiodothyronine (T3) are two thyroid hormones that are involved in the general regulation of metabolism. Although they don't directly control blood sugar, they do affect how sensitive tissues are to insulin. Thyroid hormone imbalances may be a factor in insulin resistance or a higher risk of hypoglycemia.

Ghrelin and leptin:

The hormones leptin and ghrelin are mainly linked to energy balance and appetite control. Fat cells create leptin, which alerts the brain to satiety and decreases hunger. The stomach produces ghrelin, which increases appetite. Both hormones regulate food intake and energy expenditure, which has an indirect effect on blood sugar levels.

Mechanisms of Feedback:

To keep things in balance, blood sugar management uses intricate feedback mechanisms. For instance, following a meal, increased blood glucose causes the release of insulin. Insulin lowers blood sugar levels by encouraging cells to absorb glucose. On the other hand, when blood sugar levels drop in between meals, glucagon is released and blood sugar is raised through the breakdown of glycogen and gluconeogenesis.

The Effect of Unbalances:

Several health problems can arise from improper regulation of the hormone systems that regulate blood sugar. Insulin resistance, a state in which cells lose their insulin sensitivity, frequently occurs before type 2 diabetes. Hypoglycemia (low blood sugar) and hyperglycemia (high blood sugar), both of which hurt the body's organs and systems, can also be caused by hormonal imbalances.

what distinguishes type 2 diabetes from type 1 diabetes?

Diabetes type 1 and type 2 are two different conditions with different causes, signs, and therapies. An autoimmune disease known as type 1 diabetes can strike unexpectedly and may be brought on by unknown or hereditary reasons. Little or no insulin is produced as a result of the immune system attacking and killing the pancreatic beta cells that produce insulin. Conversely, type 2 diabetes is a chronic condition for which weight and inactivity are major risk factors. Insulin resistance, a condition in which the body still generates insulin but is unable to use it efficiently, is present in people with type 2 diabetes.

Causes: Type 1 diabetes appears early in life and is thought to be the result of an autoimmune response. Over a long period, type 2 diabetes develops and is linked to lifestyle choices, including obesity and inactivity.

Type 1 diabetes symptoms include excessive thirst, frequent urination, intense hunger, unexplained weight loss, and weariness. These symptoms might appear suddenly. Type 2 diabetes can cause a variety of symptoms, such as increased thirst, frequent urination, impaired vision, sluggish wound and bruise healing, and tingling or numbness in the hands and feet.

Insulin therapy is used to treat type 1 diabetes by substituting the insulin that the body is unable to produce. Type 2 diabetes is treated with diet and activity modifications, oral medicines, and, if necessary, insulin therapy.

It's crucial to remember that both forms of diabetes can result in persistently elevated blood sugar levels, which raises the risk of complications from the disease.

How to avoid developing diabetes types 1 and 2:

Diabetes type 1 and type 2 are two different conditions with different causes, signs, and therapies. There are various strategies to lower the chance of getting type 2 diabetes, but there is no proven strategy to prevent type 1 diabetes. The following advice will assist you in avoiding Type 2 diabetes:

Keep your weight in check. One of the biggest risk factors for type 2 diabetes is being overweight or obese. Even a modest weight loss can help lower your risk.

Engage in regular exercise: Maintaining a healthy weight and lowering your risk of type 2 diabetes can be achieved through regular physical activity. Try to get in at least 150 minutes a week of moderate-to-intense activity.

Consume a balanced diet: You can lower your chance of acquiring Type 2 diabetes by eating a nutritious diet high in fruits, vegetables, and fiber, and low in refined carbohydrates and sugar.

Steer clear of smoke. Smoking increases the risk of type 2 diabetes and a host of other illnesses. Giving up smoking can lower your risk.

Make sure you get enough sleep because not getting enough sleep can raise your risk of developing type 2 diabetes. Try to get seven hours of sleep every night.

In case you have a high chance of getting Type 2 diabetes, your physician can suggest taking medication or keeping an eye on your blood sugar levels as extra precautionary measures. It's critical to discuss your risk factors with your physician and create a strategy to lower your chance of getting type 2 diabetes.

5. The Microbiota and the Gut

The intricate ecosystem that makes up the human gut is essential to preserving general health. The microbiota, a varied community of bacteria that live in the digestive tract, is the center of this complex system. The gut microbiota, which is made up of bacteria, viruses, fungi, and other microorganisms, has come under close scientific investigation because of its substantial effects on many facets of human physiology.

The Diversity and Composition of the Microbiota

The community of gut microbiota is highly active and diversified. It lives in symbiosis with the human host and is made up of trillions of bacteria. The majority of the members are bacteria, with Bacteroidetes and Firmicutes being the two most prevalent phyla. Individual differences in composition are caused by a variety of factors, including age, food, genetics, and environmental exposures.

The Gut Microbiota's Roles:

The delicate balance in the gut is dependent on the microbiota. Its effects on the immune system, metabolism, and even brain processes go well beyond digestion. These microbes assist in the digestion of complex carbohydrates, aid in the manufacture of important vitamins, and aid in the absorption of nutrients.

Impact of the Gut-Brain Axis on Mental Health

The gut-brain axis, a remarkable relationship between the gut and the brain, has been revealed by a recent study. Through a variety of signaling channels, the microbiota interacts with the central nervous system to affect mood, thought processes, and behavior. Imbalances in the gut microbiota have been linked to mental health issues, raising interest in the potential therapeutic implications of modifying the microbiome for mental well-being.

Immune System Control:

The stomach acts as a vital conduit between the body's internal environment and the outside world. The microbiome is essential for immune system education and modulation. It helps discriminate between safe antigens and dangerous infections, ensuring a proper immune response. Allergies, autoimmune illnesses, and chronic inflammation are immune-related problems that can result from disturbances in this delicate equilibrium.

Metabolic Health and Gut Microbiota

The gut microbiota is closely related to metabolic health. These microbes affect how energy is metabolized, control hunger, and help break down food into energy. An imbalance in the composition of the microbiota, known as dysbiosis, has been linked to metabolic diseases like diabetes and obesity. Comprehending these associations creates opportunities for prospective therapies aimed at the microbiota to address metabolic disorders.

Variables Affecting the Gut Microbiota

The diversity and makeup of the gut microbiota are influenced by multiple factors. Microbial populations are influenced by lifestyle choices, antibiotic use, food preferences, and environmental exposures. Antibiotics are essential for treating infections, but they can also randomly upset the delicate balance of gut microorganisms. For this reason, it's important to use them sparingly to avoid unwanted side effects.

The Potential Benefits of Changing the Microbiota

The investigation of therapeutic approaches that target the gut microbiota has resulted from the realization of the microbiota's crucial role in both health and disease. New methods are emerging to modify the microbiota for medicinal purposes, including probiotics, prebiotics, and fecal microbiota transplantation. Innovative treatments for a range of ailments, from systemic diseases to gastrointestinal issues, may result from research in this area.

Obstacles and Prospects for the Future
Even though our knowledge of the gut microbiota has grown, there are still issues. Deciphering the microbiota's various roles is complicated by the dynamic nature of the microbiota, inter-individual variability, and complexity of the microbial community. Future studies will probably concentrate on deciphering the complex gut microbiota and creating

individualized treatments based on each person's microbial composition.

There are many methods to improve gut health:
Maintain a healthy gut by eating a balanced diet that is high in fruits, vegetables, whole grains, and lean protein. Steer clear of processed foods, foods heavy in fat, and sugary drinks, as these can have a detrimental effect on gut health.
Keep your body hydrated. Eating a lot of water helps maintain a healthy digestive tract.
Engage in regular exercise: By lowering stress and encouraging regular bowel movements, regular exercise can support the maintenance of a healthy gut. A lack of sleep can have a detrimental effect on gut health, so get enough rest. Get seven to eight hours of sleep every night.

Decrease stress: Excessive stress might be detrimental to intestinal health. Try practicing stress-relieving techniques like yoga, meditation, or deep breathing.

Consider probiotics: these live bacteria can aid in reestablishing the proper balance of gut flora. They can be found in fermented foods such as yogurt, kefir, and sauerkraut or taken as supplements.

Consume foods high in prebiotics; these fibers help to nourish the beneficial bacteria in your stomach. Prebiotic-rich foods include onions, garlic, bananas, and asparagus.

Antibiotics can destroy both good and harmful bacteria in the gut, so only use them when necessary. Refrain from using antibiotics unless required.

Steer clear of smoking and excessive alcohol intake. These behaviors might have a detrimental effect on intestinal health.

6. The Intricacies of Brain Function and Neurotransmitters

The complex network of neurons, synapses, and neurotransmitters that make up the human brain is a marvel of evolution, coordinating the symphony of our feelings, ideas, and behaviors. By understanding the intricate interactions between neurotransmitters and brain activity, we can reveal the secrets of cognition and behavior.

Neurons, the basic units of the nervous system, are crucial to brain function. Synapses, which are junctions where signals are sent from one neuron to another, are how these specialized cells communicate. Neurotransmitters, chemical messengers that are essential in forming our mental environment, mediate the machinery of this exchange.

There are many different kinds of neurotransmitters, and each has a special purpose and impact on the brain. Dopamine, which is frequently linked to reward and pleasure, is one of the most well-known neurotransmitters. Dopamine is essential for motor control in addition to being a factor in motivation and pleasure. Parkinson's disease and schizophrenia have been associated with dopamine imbalances, indicating the importance of this neurotransmitter in preserving normal brain function. Another essential neurotransmitter known as the "feel-good" neurotransmitter is serotonin. It affects our emotional health by controlling our mood, hunger, and sleep patterns. Depression and anxiety are examples of mood disorders linked to changes in serotonin levels. Doctors often prescribe drugs that block serotonin receptors to treat symptoms and restore the body's equilibrium.

The neurotransmitter acetylcholine, which plays a role in memory and learning, emphasizes how crucial brain function is to cognitive functions. Acetylcholine plays a critical role in sustaining cognitive health, as seen by the deficiencies seen in illnesses such as Alzheimer's disease. Comprehending the cholinergic dynamics provides insight into the complexities involved in memory creation and retrieval.

As an inhibitory neurotransmitter, gamma-amino-butyric acid (GABA) controls brain activity and inhibits excessive neuronal firing. Abnormalities in GABA distribution link epilepsy and anxiety disorders. Neural networks require a careful balance between excitatory and inhibitory neurotransmitters to remain stable.

The main excitatory neurotransmitter in the brain, however, is glutamate. It is essential for synaptic plasticity, which is the capacity of synapses to change in strength over time. Glutamate's role in learning and memory activities makes its dysregulation a link to neurodegenerative diseases like Alzheimer's, according to researchers.

The intricate dance of neurotransmitters is a dynamic, ongoing activity rather than being limited to discrete moments. Precisely calibrated systems of neurotransmitter release, reuptake, and receptor binding ensured precise communication between neurons. Disturbances in these systems can have a domino effect on behavior, mood, and thought processes.

An imbalance of neurotransmitters can result from several things, such as lifestyle choices, environmental variables, and heredity. Using this understanding, the rapidly developing discipline of neuropharmacology aims to provide focused treatments for neurological and mental conditions. Neurotransmitter activity-modulating medications aim to balance and relieve symptoms, offering a glimmer of hope to people struggling with mental health issues.

Researchers in various fields, including pharmacology, psychology, neurology, and psychiatry, can explore beyond the study of neurotransmitters. Research on neurotransmitters has made it possible to comprehend how the brain shapes our experiences and perceptions on a deeper level. With the development of technology, neuroimaging methods have opened up new avenues for our study of the mind by enabling us to watch, in real-time, the complex dance of neurotransmitters.

PART 3

Nourishing Habits: A Guide on How to Eat to Modify Your Drinking

The importance of the interaction between our lifestyle choices and food choices cannot be overstated in our pursuit of total well-being. Alcohol use is one such lifestyle factor that frequently needs to be changed. Eating with awareness can have a big influence on our drinking patterns. This article examines the complex relationship between alcohol consumption and nutrition, providing information on how a healthy diet can be the cornerstone of positive lifestyle modifications.

Recognizing the connection:
It is important to recognize the role that nutrients play in impacting our physical and mental moods to understand the relationship between eating habits and drinking behavior. Foods high in nutrients promote mental clarity and emotional stability, serving as a protective barrier against the harmful consequences of binge drinking. Maintaining a constant blood sugar level is supported by maintaining a balance of macronutrients, which include proteins, fats, and carbohydrates. This lessens the chance of energy swings that could lead to rash choices, including binge drinking. Make whole grains, lean proteins, and healthy fats your top priorities if you want to have continuous energy all day.

Minerals and vitamins: Proper consumption of minerals and vitamins is necessary for several physiological functions, including mood control. A lack of some nutrients may make people more likely to turn to alcohol for comfort. A wide range of vital vitamins and minerals can be obtained by eating a variety of fruits, vegetables, and whole meals.

Useful Advice for Adjustment:

Mindful Eating: Practicing mindfulness while eating raises awareness of signs of hunger and fullness. People can lessen the chance of using alcohol as a coping method for stress or emotional discomfort by enjoying every bite and paying attention to their bodies' cues.

Hydration: Maintaining proper hydration is essential for general health and may have little influence on drinking patterns. The body may occasionally mistake thirst for an alcohol urge. Throughout the day, sipping water can help you stay hydrated and lessen your desire to seek out alcohol.

Timing Your Meals Strategically: Arrange your meals to take place at times when people might be drinking. Before social gatherings, when alcohol is served, having a well-balanced lunch can help reduce the amount of alcohol absorbed and lessen its immediate effects. Add healthy fats and proteins to reinforce this tactic.

Nutrient-Dense Snacking: When cravings strike, choose nutrient-dense foods. Fruits, nuts, and seeds are a filling substitute for high-calorie snacks and may also reduce the urge to drink. These snacks enhance general well-being by adding nutrition to the diet.

The Function of Particular Foods: Omega-3 Fatty Acids: Linked to better mood and cognitive performance, omega-3 fatty acids are found in walnuts, flaxseeds, and fatty fish. By including these foods in your diet, you may be able to maintain a more upbeat emotional state and lessen your dependency on alcohol to improve your mood.

Complex carbs: Foods high in complex carbs, such as whole grains, legumes, and vegetables, help produce serotonin, a neurotransmitter linked to positive emotions. A steady level of serotonin may reduce the need to turn to alcohol for solace.

Adopting a holistic approach that incorporates mindful eating and a well-balanced diet is essential in the quest to change drinking habits. People can establish healthier choices by being aware of the complex relationship between nutrition and mental health. The process of changing one's drinking habits is not just about abstaining; it's also about taking advantage of opportunities to support mental and physical well-being and develop a positive, long-lasting lifestyle. Recall that gradual modifications in eating patterns can have a big impact on general well-being and have a good long-term effect on drinking habits.

7. Begin Where You Are

The journey of life is a never-ending stream of events and time. We are often faced with circumstances that require us to make choices that will have an impact on our future. "Starting Where You Are" offers simple yet sage advice that is highly relevant in these times. It encapsulates an idea that stresses accepting oneself and one's circumstances while simultaneously making the initial move toward a better tomorrow.

Life can feel overwhelming sometimes because of how complicated it is. Self-imposed norms, social pressures, and constant comparison to others can all contribute to feelings of insecurity and anxiety about oneself. "Starting Where You Are" offers a respite from this chaos by urging us to firmly establish ourselves in the reality of the present moment. It promotes introspection and assists us in evaluating our benefits, drawbacks, objectives, and concerns.

Making a self-awareness assessment of oneself is a crucial step in the process of personal development. It demands an honest assessment of our current capabilities, resources, and viewpoints. When we are self-aware, it becomes a compass that guides our decisions and actions. We focus on the specific steps we can take right now, rather than letting the vastness of our goals immobilize us. The concept of "Starting Where You Are" does not downplay the importance of goals or the future. Instead, it's about creating a workable roadmap that considers the conditions of the world we already live in. This approach promotes agency, enabling us to take command of our lives and make deliberate choices. It creates a proactive mentality in which difficulties are perceived as opportunities for progress and failures as learning experiences.

One of the fundamental tenets of starting where you are is accepting your imperfections. Perfectionism's impossible standards can be a debilitating influence. When we acknowledge that every individual starts from a different location and encounters unique challenges and circumstances, we are set free from the bonds of perfection. It provides access to growth, education, and the fortitude required to face life's uncertainties. Additionally, "Starting Where You Are" exhorts listeners to live in the now. It's easy to become bogged down in regrets about the past or anxieties about the future. However, this is the moment when we may make positive changes. By embracing the moment as it is, we may focus on worthwhile activities. Being aware enhances our capacity for decision-making and generally makes life more pleasurable.

The concept applies to many aspects of society and is not just restricted to the personal realm. Organizations can utilize this idea, for instance, to assess their existing condition, pinpoint their advantages and disadvantages, and develop long-term strategic strategies. It promotes a culture of continuous improvement where inventiveness and adaptability are essential for success.

In partnerships, the idea of "Starting Where You Are" fosters compassion and understanding. It fosters an understanding that growth is a shared experience among friends, family, and partners, encouraging respect for one another's unique origins. This approach creates a supportive environment where people can grow without fear of criticism. There are other benefits to this way of thinking about schooling. Recognizing the diverse starting points of students allows for a more comprehensive and individualized approach to teaching. It accepts the idea that each person, regardless of their upbringing, possesses special abilities and potential.

"Starting Where You Are" is a notion that encapsulates the essence of personal and collective growth. It reminds us that all it takes is one step to go a thousand miles, and the best place to start is right now, where you are. By acknowledging our inadequacies, being present, and living in the present, we create space for a future shaped by conscious choices and unwavering progress

8. A 4-Week Dietary and Nutrition Plan to Reduce Your Drinking

Drinking too much alcohol can be harmful to one's physical and emotional well-being. A balanced nutrition and food plan can be quite helpful in helping people who want to cut back on their alcohol consumption. To enhance general well-being, the emphasis of this 4-week strategy is on combining nutrient-rich foods, hydration techniques, and mindful eating habits.

Week 1: Refueling and Elimination of Toxins

To kickstart the trip, prioritize staying hydrated. Increase water intake to eliminate toxins from the body and improve liver function. For extra taste and health advantages, try adding infused water and herbal teas. Antioxidant-rich foods, including citrus fruits, leafy greens, and berries, help with detoxification. Start cutting back on sugar-filled drinks and processed meals to promote a healthy lifestyle.

Week 2: foods high in nutrients

Place a focus on nutrient-dense foods that are rich in important minerals and vitamins. Add nutritious grains, lean proteins, and a rainbow of vibrant vegetables. Walnuts, flaxseeds, and fatty fish are good sources of omega-3 fatty acids, which can help with brain function and lessen cravings. Arrange well-balanced meals to prevent blood sugar surges that could lead to cravings for alcohol.

Week 3: Modifying Behavior and Mindful Eating

Increase your awareness of hunger and satiety hicues by engaging in mindful eating. During meals, take your time, enjoy every bite, and be mindful of the portion proportions. Determine the factors that contribute to binge drinking and create alternate coping mechanisms. Reduce your dependency on alcohol by managing your emotional well-being by incorporating stress-relieving hobbies like yoga or meditation.

Week 4: Probiotics and Gut Health

In addition to improving general health, a healthy gut can affect desires. To improve gut health, include foods high in probiotics, such as kefir, yogurt, and fermented vegetables. Whole grains and legumes are examples of foods high in fiber that improve digestion and help control blood sugar levels. Consuming enough fiber also makes you feel fuller and less likely to reach for booze when you're uncomfortable.

Continuous Approaches:

Frequent Physical Activity: Exercise regularly to improve mood, relieve stress, and give positive vent to feelings that could lead to alcohol use.

Social Support: Make sure you have a strong support system of friends and family around you. Share your objectives and look for support from others who are aware of your trip.

Specialist Advice: To customize the strategy to your unique needs and address underlying concerns, think about consulting with a nutritionist, dietitian, or mental health specialist.

Ongoing Education: Remain up-to-date on the effects of diet on general health. Knowing the link between health and nutrition helps strengthen healthy behaviors.

Through addressing the behavioral, emotional, and physical components of alcohol usage, this 4-week dietary and nutrition plan seeks to provide a holistic approach to alcohol reduction. A balanced lifestyle that incorporates meals high in nutrients, plenty of water, mindfulness, and continuing support can help people develop and sustain a better relationship with alcohol over the long run.

9. Supplements, Herbs, and Other Modifications to Lifestyle

People are using vitamins, herbs, and lifestyle changes to improve their general health in a society where wellness has become a top priority. The drive to proactively manage health, stave off diseases, and enhance performance is what's driving this change. This article examines the wide range of supplements available, the effectiveness of herbs, and the effects of changing our lifestyle on our mental and physical well-being.

Supplements: Filling Up the Nutrient Gaps

Because they provide a practical solution for correcting nutritional inadequacies in our modern diets, supplements have become increasingly popular. From critical vitamins like Vitamin C and D to minerals such as iron and magnesium, supplements operate as a safety net to ensure our bodies acquire the necessary elements for optimal function. But it's important to be cautious when supplementing because taking too much of it can have negative effects. Speaking with medical experts can assist in customizing supplement regimens to meet specific requirements, guaranteeing a well-rounded and unique approach to nutritional support.

Herbs: Nature's Prescription

Herbs have been a part of many traditional medical procedures around the world for ages. Their all-natural ingredients provide a comprehensive approach to wellness, treating underlying imbalances as well as symptoms. Herbs that are proven to reduce inflammation include ginger and turmeric, while chamomile and valerian roots help promote calmness and sleep. It's important to be aware of the qualities of herbs and any potential drug interactions before incorporating them into daily practice. Harnessing the medicinal properties of plants efficiently requires striking a balance between tradition and scientific data.

Modifications to Lifestyle: Establishing a Basis for Well-Being

Lifestyle changes are crucial in determining our general health, even in addition to vitamins and herbs. The cornerstones of a healthy lifestyle include adequate sleep, stress management, a balanced diet, and regular exercise. By forming these routines, one can avoid a wide range of health problems, including mental and cardiovascular difficulties. But changing one's lifestyle demands dedication and a steady, step-by-step approach. Less drastic, short-term fixes frequently result in more significant long-term advantages than small, continuous adjustments.

Personalization in Health: A Customized Method

When it comes to well-being and health, there is no one-size-fits-all solution. Everybody's body reacts differently to various medicines, vitamins, and lifestyle adjustments. The secret to realizing these interventions' full potential is personalization. Our bodies' responses to different wellness initiatives are influenced by a combination of genetic factors, pre-existing health issues, and lifestyle choices. With the development of technology, people may now more easily access customized nutrition and wellness programs, enabling them to make decisions based on their specific profiles.

Difficulties and debates

There are still issues and disagreements surrounding supplements, herbs, and lifestyle changes, even with the increased interest in them. Concerns regarding the safety and quality of supplements are raised by the absence of strict regulations in this sector. Furthermore, inconsistent data about the effectiveness of particular herbs and supplements may cause misunderstandings among buyers. To manage potential hazards, it is crucial to approach these therapies with caution, depending on information based on evidence and speaking with medical professionals.

The relationship between the mind and body

In the quest for holistic wellness, the complex interrelationship between the mind and body cannot be disregarded. Complementing the physical components addressed by vitamins and herbs, mental and emotional well-being is enhanced by practices such as yoga, mindfulness, and meditation. Acknowledging and promoting the mind-body link promotes a holistic approach to health that goes beyond physical exercise.

Forward-Looking: Integrative Medicine

The idea of integrative medicine arises as the lines separating traditional and complementary care become more blurred. This method recognizes the importance of a holistic approach to health and integrates evidence-based techniques from both fields. Integrative medicine promotes teamwork among medical specialists and gives patients the freedom to consider a variety of solutions for their health. The key to wellness in the future is to embrace diversity and keep learning more about how different interventions work together to promote good health.

10.   Building Strong Communities: The Foundation of a Thriving Society

It is impossible to overestimate the significance of building and maintaining strong communities in a world of rapid change. A community is a dynamic network of people who have similar interests, values, and aspirations, rather than just being a collection of people who live in the same place. Building a healthy community involves more than just

setting up a physical location; it also entails developing relationships, a sense of community, and cooperation among its constituents.

Recognizing the Fundamental Nature of Community:

Any society is built on its communities, which act as a network of support for individuals and a fertile ground for the exchange of common experiences. Communities provide people with a sense of purpose, stability, and identity, whether they live in an urban or rural area. They are essential in forming people's lives, impacting their well-being, and strengthening the social fabric as a whole.

The Basis of Confidence:

Trust is the foundation of any successful community. Establishing mutual respect, open communication, and transparency are all important components of the complex process of building trust among community members. People are more likely to actively participate, contribute, and collaborate in their community when they feel safe and encouraged, which creates an atmosphere People here, everyone may flourish.

Building Inclusive Environments: Establishing welcoming and inclusive environments is essential to community formation. from different origins, ethnicities, and viewpoints are welcomed into an inclusive community that values the strength that comes from the diversity of viewpoints and experiences. Members of the community benefit from this inclusivity by developing empathy and understanding, as well as a rich tapestry of ideas.

Interaction and Communication: Any community needs effective communication to survive. By creating open lines of communication, members may remain informed and involved since information can flow easily. Furthermore, developing deep ties within the community enhances general well-being by establishing a sense of belonging and lowering feelings of loneliness.

Common Purposes and Ideals:
Common aims and ideals form the cornerstone of any thriving community. These guiding ideals give the community direction and a sense of purpose, pointing it in the direction of constructive development. When members of a community work together toward a similar goal, they generate a strong force that can overcome obstacles and succeed as a group.

Cooperation and self-determination:
When people feel encouraged to share their abilities, communities flourish. A sense of pride and ownership is fostered by promoting teamwork and giving participants the chance to actively engage in decision-making processes.

Empowered individuals are more inclined to take initiative, generate constructive change, and contribute to the general betterment of the community.

Flexibility and Sturdiness:
In a world that is continuously changing, communities need to be resilient and adaptive. Long-term sustainability requires the capacity to deal with change, overcome obstacles, and draw lessons from failures. Giving a community's members the means to triumph over misfortune while preserving their sense of solidarity is a key component in building resilience.

Civic Leadership:
A community's leadership is essential to directing its development and growth. Effective leaders listen to the needs of community members, promote collaboration, and work for the common good. Inclusionary leadership should promote a culture of continual

improvement, support a range of viewpoints, and encourage participation. Advantages of a Robust Community: Numerous advantages accrue not only to the individuals within a strong community but also to society as a whole. These include a stronger sense of security, better mental health, higher civic involvement, and improved social well-being. Furthermore, socially cohesive groups are better able to deal with problems that affect the whole community, such as environmental issues and economic downturns.

Creating and maintaining a thriving community is a team effort that calls for cooperation, dedication, and communication. In addition to reflecting the people who live there, a vibrant community catalyzes constructive change in society at large. By acknowledging the significance of trust, inclusivity, shared values, and cooperation, we may

establish the groundwork for
communities that promote resilience,
empower individuals, and enhance the
overall welfare of their constituents. The
resilience of our communities will always
be essential to a vibrant, globalized
society as we all continue to change and
grow.

PART 4
Recipes

11.   Nourishing Recipes for a Healthier You: Supporting Your Alcohol Reduction Plan

Starting a journey to cut back on drinking is a noble endeavor that enhances general well-being. One crucial component of this process is choosing a nutritious and balanced diet that not only promotes your body's recuperation but also adds to your mental and physical wellness. We'll look at several dishes in this article that fit into your alcohol reduction plan and will provide you with tasty options that are good for your body and mind.

Smoothies Packed with Vegetables: To speed up your metabolism, start your day with a smoothie that's high in nutrients. To make a tasty and satisfying drink, blend kale, spinach, berries, banana, and a scoop of protein powder. Your body will be detoxified by the antioxidants in the berries, as well as the vitamins and minerals in the leafy greens.

Quinoa Salad with Fresh Veggies: A substantial salad can be built around the versatile and protein-rich grain known as quinoa. Toss cooked quinoa with vibrant veggies such as bell peppers, cucumbers, and cherry tomatoes, then drizzle with a mild vinaigrette dressing. This hearty salad gives you the fiber and other vital elements you need to be full and energized.

Baked Salmon with Lemon and **Herbs:** Baked salmon is a delicious way to get omega-3 fatty acids into your diet. Add some lemon juice, fresh herbs, and a little olive oil to season it. In addition to providing nutrients like vitamin D, which is essential for general well-being, salmon also promotes heart health. Stuffed Chicken Breast with **Mushroom and Spinach:** Choose lean protein sources, such as chicken breast, and stuff them with a blend of sautéed mushrooms and spinach. This dish is a pleasant and nutritious substitute for heavier, alcohol-pairing meals because it is high in protein, vitamins, and minerals.

Sweet Potato and Chickpea Curry: Try making a curry using sweet potatoes and chickpeas as a plant-based supper. This delectable recipe helps you achieve your nutritional goals while satisfying your taste buds. It is packed with fiber, protein, and other vitamins.

Greek Yogurt Parfait: Top Greek yogurt with almonds, fresh fruit, and a honey drizzle for a guilt-free snack or dessert. Probiotics and protein are abundant in Greek yogurt, which also happens to be a delicious and filling dessert.

Green Tea-Infused Quenchers: Try these cool tea infusions instead of sweetened drinks. Combine cucumber, mint, and citrus slices to create a refreshing beverage that is high in antioxidants. Additionally, green tea can help increase metabolism and improve general health.

Whole Grain Pasta with Tomato and **Basil Sauce:** If you're looking for a high-fiber substitute for regular pasta, try whole-grain pasta. For a fresh and wholesome dinner that fulfills your needs for pasta without sacrificing your health objectives, top it with a homemade tomato and basil sauce.

12.   The World of Mocktails and Tonics

In recent times, mocktails and tonics have gained popularity as a refreshing, non-alcoholic substitute for classic cocktails. Those seeking tasty, stimulating drinks without the hangover consequences of alcohol have welcomed this trend. In this note, we will explore the history, variety of tastes, and techniques of creating these delectable drinks as we dig into the realm of mocktails and tonics.

History and Origins: Mocktails, often known as "mock cocktails," have been around for several years, developing throughout time from straightforward fruit juice mixtures to complex, well-balanced drinks. Mocktails are becoming more and more popular, which is indicative of a shift in public views toward a more aware and health-conscious way of living and the growing need for non-alcoholic options. Conversely, tonics were historically defined as carbonated water flavored with quinine and frequently combined with gin. But the phrase now refers to a broad variety of non-alcoholic drinks that share the same effervescent characteristics.

Ingredients and Flavor Profiles: The variety of ingredients used to generate distinctive and pleasing flavor profiles is one of the interesting characteristics of mocktails and tonics. These mixtures often contain fresh fruits, herbs, syrups, and different infusions. The choices are boundless, ranging from the earthy undertones of a tonic steeped with lavender to the zesty citrus notes of a virgin mojito. These drinks provide a delightful experience for the palate, demonstrating that alcohol is not necessary to enjoy a sophisticated and savory drink.

Making the Ideal Mocktail: A harmonious combination of flavors, textures, and scents is necessary to create the ideal mocktail. Professional and amateur mixologists alike have taken on the challenge of crafting mocktails with the intricacy and allure of their alcoholic counterparts. A big part of improving the entire drinking experience is mastering the techniques of garnishing, shaking, and muddling. The desire for creatively made mocktails has prompted an interesting expansion in the field of non-alcoholic mixology as customers look for more thoughtful options.

Impact on Society and Culture: Mocktails and tonics have not only established themselves as standard fare in pubs and restaurants, but they have also left their stamp on society and cultural gatherings. These drinks, which range from sober celebrations to alcohol-free brunches, are dispelling the stigma attached to abstaining from alcohol. For those who abstain from alcohol due to health concerns, personal preferences, or to act as a designated driver, they offer inclusive solutions. This culture change is a reflection of a wider acceptance of different lifestyles and the value of providing options that satisfy everyone. **Health and Wellness:** Mocktails and tonics, aside from their delicious flavor, add to the increasing focus on health and wellness. As people become more conscious of the possible drawbacks of binge drinking, a growing number of them choose non-alcoholic substitutes that complement their health objectives. These drinks' vivid hues and freshly squeezed ingredients provide a visual feast that heightens the senses as a whole.

Conclusion

Drinking habits can be greatly impacted and modified by taking a thoughtful and deliberate approach to nutrition. People can lower their risk of excessive alcohol intake and promote their well-being by making informed decisions based on their awareness of how food and alcohol interact.

An important thing to think about is how nutrient-dense meals affect how the body processes alcohol. Eating a healthy, vitamin- and mineral-rich diet high in antioxidants helps improve liver function and helps with the detoxification process. This benefits general health as well as improving the body's ability to metabolize alcohol, which may lessen the harmful consequences of binge drinking.

Additionally, a key factor in reducing alcohol use is the timing of meals. Eating before consuming alcohol lessens its immediate effects by delaying the bloodstream's absorption of the alcohol. Selecting meals that are high in a combination of healthy fats, proteins, and carbs can provide people with a steady energy boost and help them better regulate how much alcohol they drink during parties or social occasions. Hydration is yet another important factor. Maintaining proper hydration levels can be facilitated by including foods high in water, like fruits and vegetables, in the diet. Maintaining adequate hydration helps lessen the drying effects of alcohol while also supporting general health. Maintaining adequate hydration levels can enhance the pleasure of alcohol consumption and lower the risk of overindulging in alcohol.

Understanding the link between drinking patterns and emotional health is crucial. Unhealthy patterns can be produced by emotional eating or drinking in reaction to stress, worry, or other emotions. The pattern of utilizing food or alcohol as a coping method for emotions can be broken by embracing alternate coping strategies like exercise, mindfulness, or asking friends and family for assistance. It's also critical to pay attention to alcohol content and meal proportions. One of the most important parts of maintaining a healthy lifestyle is managing how much food and drink you consume. An approach to eating and drinking that is more sustainable and balanced can be achieved by recognizing one's own boundaries and establishing reasonable goals for moderation.

It takes a diversified strategy to change drinking behaviors through food. It includes knowing the effects of diet on the metabolism of alcohol, planning meals strategically, staying hydrated, maintaining mental stability, and controlling portion sizes. People can cultivate a better relationship with alcohol and improve their physical and mental health by adopting these lifestyle practices.

There is no one-size-fits-all approach to changing drinking habits; it is ultimately a personal journey. It calls for self-awareness, dedication, and the readiness to make wise decisions. Consulting with medical specialists or nutritionists can offer tailored counsel and encouragement on integrating these concepts into a person's particular way of life. A proactive, all-encompassing approach to nutrition can enable people to take charge of their health, make good changes, and develop more harmonious, satisfying relationships with food and alcohol.

www.ingramcontent.com/pod-product-compliance
Lightning Source LLC
Chambersburg PA
CBHW071608270726
48661CB00019B/1657